Vedda Blood Sugar Remedy

Kevin Donohue

Copyright © 2018 Kevin Donohue

All rights reserved.

ISBN: 9781980484929

CONTENTS

1. WHAT IS DIABETES? — 3
2. WHAT SHOULD YOU KNOW ABOUT VEDDA BLOOD SUGAR REMEDY — 9
3. The 30-Day Schedule to Reduce the Sugar Level in Your Blood — 24
4. HIIT – THE WEAPON TO FIGHT DIABETES — 43
5. Blood Sugar Lowering Smoothies — 52
6. CONCLUSION — 73

Readers are highly recommended to seek proper advice from either a physician or a professional practitioner before implementing any of these suggestions. Seriously, this book cannot replace professional and medical advice. Therefore, both the author and the publisher will not take any responsibility for any adverse results if readers really follow the information herein.

I. Introduction

Vedda Blood Sugar Remedy is a great book! It is going to give you a clear overview of diabetes including type I and type II, which are considered as one of the most common lethal diseases these days.

As you may know, you cannot get rid of diabetes with the recent technology. Instead, thanks to the dietary strategies which come from a group of people living in Sri Lanka, you can gradually overcome diabetes.

As a result, this book is going to help you learn the basics on how to find the best solutions to this disease by knowing our ancestors' lifestyle patterns, as well as applying for the popular HIIT training program.

Moreover, in case you are suffering from high blood pressure, you are advised to meet with your doctors to discuss possible medication and any medical related issues. By consulting with your doctors, you can get better results day by day.

In general, you can greatly decrease the chances of getting diabetes when strictly applying the useful strategies mentioned in this book. Also, this book will present the potential problems for anyone having high blood pressure. You will have a chance to learn the entire process of how to lower your blood sugar level.

Each part of this book is written based on my real-life experience, together with other well-known health specialists all around the world.

Finally, make sure you can really enjoy your life when reading every page of this book. I hope you can understand why we need to live healthily by trying to eliminate diabetes after going through all the chapters of this book. It is a very challenging process, but really deserves your efforts. Thanks for reading this book and best luck to you!

II. CHAPTER I: WHAT IS DIABETES?

What is diabetes?

These days, many people are enduring the effects of diabetes resulting from their unhealthy living standards and eating habits. Based on the statistics from the International Diabetes Federation, there are over 387 million cases of diabetes at this moment. Also, this number does not have a decreasing tendency, but is expected to go up to 592 million by 2035. More seriously, every 7 seconds one person is reported to die of diabetes.

With all these details, we are facing a very alarming issue. So, do you know what diabetes is?

Firstly, diabetes exists when your body is gradually losing the ability to produce as well as respond to the hormone insulin. If there is a lack of insulin, your body can't regulate the level of glucose in the blood. This will result in an imbalanced concentration of glucose, and unluckily, this is considered as the main form of sugar.

In general, glucose is known as the key source of energy for our body and our body needs this element. It comes from many things that we eat every day.

Moreover, there are many types of diabetes that you should know such as type I, type II, pre-diabetes, gestational diabetes and latent autoimmune diabetes. We will discuss all of them in detail when moving onto the next part.

Types of diabetes

Diabetes type I and II are the two most common ones. So, let's get to know them better!

Normally, type I and type II diabetes are certainly the most well-known, and now we are going to identify more information about them.

You can also call type I diabetes idiopathic or immune-mediated diabetes. Young people have a higher chance to have this type, which destroys the beta cells in the Islets of Langerhans areas. These beta cells can produce insulin, which helps our body to convert glucose into energy. Therefore, if they cannot work properly, the sugar extracted from the food will either remain in your blood or pass into the urine.

There are several symptoms to let you realize you may have type I diabetes:

- Lose weight significantly and suddenly
- Tend to feel tired more frequently
- Your vision is getting bad
- Have headaches
- Your skin is infected
- Feel weaker and dizzier
- Excessive urination
- Feel extremely thirsty constantly

Going on to type II diabetes, it is more common than type1 and tends to occur in an older group to those who are 45 and above. If you have this type, there is insufficient insulin produced by the pancreas, which leads to excess amounts of sugar remaining in your blood.

Therefore, the cells can't get access to the adequate glucose, which in turns makes your body feel fatigued and weak. Moreover, this condition will become worse since the pancreas is going to lose its ability to produce insulin and may result in causing fatal cases in the long run.

When you have type II diabetes, some of the following situations may appear:

- Excess of urination
- Extreme thirst constantly
- Cuts and wounds heal slowly
- Uncontrolled hunger
- Leg cramps and unclear vision
- Significant weight gain
- Have skin infections

Apart from these two most common types, there are other ones, including Gestational Diabetes Mellitus (GDM), Pre-diabetes and Latent autoimmune diabetes in adults (LADA.).

Gestational Diabetes Mellitus is very similar to type II diabetes and it affects pregnant women. Of course, it is not good for the health of the mothers-to-be. But luckily, the women can be treated during their pregnancies to treat the GDM through medical treatment combined with professional advice during the dangerous period. GDM usually resolves after the birth of the baby, but in some cases may not go away.

Pre-diabetes is another type of diabetes when the sugar level in your blood is excessive. However, it is not as high as in type II diabetes. Thus, people with type II diabetes usually go through a pre-diabetes stage first, which can change into type 2 diabetes in the run.

LADA shares some identical elements with type I diabetes. Besides, the development time of this type is pretty slow. Many people confuse this with type II since they also have some similar factors and symptoms.

Cause of diabetes

Until now, there are only ambiguous causes of type I and type II diabetes. Especially, some factors including your family history, your age, as well as your ethnic background, can have a great influence on developing type II diabetes. Hence, you will have a higher chance of developing diabetes if a family member has this disease.

Particularly, when you have any of these listed problems, you are more likely to develop diabetes:

- High blood pressure
- Overweight
- Does not regularly exercise
- Have improper diet process
- Inherit the genes from the family members who have this disease
- Over 45 and acquire one of the above issues
- Over 55

How diabetes impacts the health

When you have type I diabetes, **Diabetic ketoacidosis** is one of the most common effects. You will go through a disorder of the metabolism, which will lead to many serious issues such as vomiting, nausea, abdominal pain, and breathing difficulties.

Kussmaul breathing seems to happen during the diabetic ketoacidosis. It is related to deep breathing, as well as the odor of acetone appears in your breath.

Moreover, you might have to put up with **Hyperosmolar non-ketonic.** Because of the dehydration diabetics face, you may have this issue with type II diabetes.

Last but not least, **blood vessels** become the part of the body with the most dangerous impact on diabetes patients. Diabetics can develop fatal cases due to their coronary artery condition. Also, the danger in bad blood vessels can affect your nerves, your vision, and your kidneys.

The disadvantages of conventional medication

Usually, diabetes patients tend to get the proper prescribed medical treatment from their doctors. Nevertheless, nothing is better than a proper dietary habit, as well as getting frequent exercise. The reason for this advice is because people with diabetes usually have a very unhealthy eating habit and bad lifestyle. Also, you may face many unexpected side effects when taking the medication for type II diabetes.

You cannot cure type II diabetes permanently if you really have it. You need to take Metformin, which is a very excellent medication for regulating the sugar level in your blood. Despite its benefit, you must think about the side effects when taking this meditation for a long time.

For instance, you may get dizzy, endure digestive issues, as well as have sinus infections. Furthermore, Metformin is reported to greatly decrease the number of necessary B12 vitamins inside your body. Therefore, you may obtain a higher chance of heart attacks and some cardiovascular diseases.

Except for Metformin, there are other drugs used to cure diabetes. You can take Sulfonylureas, Alpha-glucosidase Inhibitors, Meglitinides, Biguanides, Thiazolidinediones, as well as DPP-4 Inhibitors. In fact, these medications cannot permanently eliminate diabetes and you can be affected by their side effects.

As a result, the easiest and simplest way is to have a good eating plan and maintain a habit of getting exercise regularly.

If you want to discover how to cure this disease effectively, the next part will give you a clear answer. I am immersed in this topic since my family members have endured it for a long time. I always try to read as many books and articles as possible. Hence, moving on to the next part, I am going to show you my real-life knowledge, along with my experience on how to treat this illness in the best way.

III. CHAPTER II: WHAT SHOULD YOU KNOW ABOUT VEDDA BLOOD SUGAR REMEDY

If you are a victim of diabetes, you might be familiar with the phrase 'Vedda blood sugar remedy'. It has earned a great reputation as being the most upgraded and effective way to cure diabetes, especially those who are fighting type II diabetes.

Reading this chapter will give you an insight on this amazing treatment which comes from the Vedda people. Make sure you go through to the end, so you may find out the proper solutions for yourself.

Vedda Origin

Do you know what the origin of Vedda is? We need to have a look at their culture, so we can deeply understand their dietary strategy. Amazingly, this group has never had ta diabetes patient. Therefore, we get to dig deep into their living habits to understand their secret.

For those people who don't know, the Vedda are the inhabitants of Sri Lanka, who are popular for being the late generations of their Neolithic ancestors. In particular, there are three main groups living separately in the Vedda, including Anuradhapura Veddas, Coast Veddas together with Bintenne Veddas.

The main task of the Vedda is hunting with the use of primitive weapons. The men will take advantage of bow and arrows, as well as using toxic plants to kill the wild animals. Moreover, the Vedda communicate with each other in a very special language. And, you will find their worship system very interesting as well.

The Vedda Dietary Habits

You must know that the meals of the Vedda are very rich in meat. After hunting, they eat animals such as fish, rabbits, turtle, venison, and even lizards. Moreover, they are very interested in a food named Gona perume, which is described as a kind of sausage with the combination of fat and alternating meat.

Furthermore, the Vedda love goya-telperume, which includes the tail of the lizard and the fat layers. Another favorite dish for the Vedda is dried meat absorbed into honey.

General Understanding

The Vedda are reported to have been living in the Sri Lanka area for a very long time. Their key physical activities are fishing, hunting and growing crops. Therefore, their daily meal consists of a large amount of protein that comes from the killed animals.

Living in the jungles, the Vedda can make full use of the fruits and vegetables, so they can always have the fibers and vitamins they need for their meals. These elements make their eating habit very ideal and similar to what the health specialists expect from people who are free from diabetes.

To prevent type II diabetes, you need to keep the sugar level in your blood at a balanced rate. So, you need to eat foods rich in protein, fiber, and healthy fat to have the best results.

You need to know that protein, fiber, and healthy fat can keep your blood sugar at a safe level. However, you need to avoid consuming excessive carbs and sugar since they are very dangerous for your health.

Moreover, you are highly recommended to eat foods that contain large amounts of the mineral chromium. In particular, broccoli is an excellent example in this case. Furthermore, consuming magnesium can do a good job in maintaining your blood sugar. For instance, beef, seeds, and nuts, as well as the vegetables are very good at providing the needed nutrients to help prevent diabetes.

As mentioned before, fiber is an amazing element to help you fight against diabetes. Besides, coconut oil is considered as the greatest treatment since it can burn fat, as well as help to balance your blood sugar level.

Apart from these factors, you need to have sufficient amounts of protein. And of course, salmon, and chicken, together with beef contain brilliant protein supplies for your body.

What Should You Look for to Eliminate the Diabetes?

Coconut

I cannot deny that coconuts are one of the most fantastic fruits that we can have in the world. This fruit can make your body healthy and vigorous. The Vedda people show much interest in coconuts, so they like putting its pulp and its milk into the food they eat.

According to the scientists, coconuts can better your health and extend your longevity. Thus, people appreciate this fruit a lot. However, most people have not known about the magical benefits of coconuts. They can be a great treatment for you to fight against diabetes.

Moreover, you can use coconut oil to prevent both the bacteria and the viruses from attacking your body. In addition, this kind of oil cannot only protect people from having cancer or heart attacks, but it also improves your skin quality and burns more fat off your body.

You must know that coconut fiber is very excellent at reducing the sugar level in your blood. Diabetics, as well as pre-diabetics, are highly suggested to consume food which does not have a high glycemic index. The reason is that this element might be one of the causes of diabetes.

When your body recognizes any signature of a high blood sugar level, it will automatically add more insulin to your blood. And coconut oil can have a great effect here. It can prevent the sugar from absorbing into your body so that your blood sugar level will be kept at a balanced rate. Another benefit of coconut oil is to reinforce blood circulation inside your body.

To be honest, coconut oil is more useful and effective than any other types of oil in terms of diabetes treatment. It can greatly reverse the bad effects that you are suffering as a result of diabetes, as well as enhance the safe rate of blood sugar in your body.

If your blood sugar is in danger after eating some kinds of food, a small amount of coconut oil will be your best solution. With no doubt, your blood sugar will be back to the safe level in only thirty minutes.

Cinnamon

The second option for your diabetes treatment is cinnamon. It is a popular spice that can make your dishes more flavorful. Moreover, you can stop your blood sugar level from elevating too much by consuming it. If you use it for a long time, the blood sugar level in your body will be less sensitive to foods.

In general, the body of the diabetic tends to reject insulin while the bodies of other people do not. This is considered as insulin resistance. However, you know that insulin is very important for everyone since it helps to release the sugar from your blood and then add it to the body cells.

When the insulin cannot get into the cells inside your body, it will cause a problem for your health. People who are enduring high blood pressure will have a higher rate of blindness. Furthermore, you can have many negative effects related to the nerves of your limbs, as well as other parts of your body.

Consequently, cinnamon is regarded as a beneficial factor to help increase your body's ability to react to insulin. The statistics in December 2003 stated that the diabetes patients had a significant decrease in blood glucose after being treated with cinnamon.

Neem

From the past until now, the Neem tree has been very popular for effectively curing several diseases. This tree can be found in the forests of Sri Lanka, and for various years, the Vedda have been using the leaves of this tree to treat a total of 40 diseases.

When talking about Neem trees, antioxidants, as well as the cancer treatment, are considered as two of their best features. In addition, this tree can do a very great job of lowering the insulin within your body only by triggering the beta cells in the pancreas.

Ginger

Going to ginger, its root is very famous for not only treating digestive problems, but also improving your overall health. Hence, your risks of having diabetes will be much lower. Until now, we have not had a clear explanation why ginger can reduce the negative condition of diabetes, but it is truly a good ingredient for your wellness.

Also, you can prevent yourselves from having other diseases when eating ginger on a regular basis. It is very great for improving arthritis, cancer, along with several cardiovascular issues.

Some Important Minerals to Prevent the Diabetes

Chromium

The first anti-diabetes mineral is chromium, which is the combination of d-nicotinic acid, chromium 3 and glutathione. This substance is also known as the Glucose Tolerance Factor that is quite similar to insulin. This mineral can be transferred from the outside to the inside of your body. Thus, diabetes can result from the improper working of chromium.

Chromium enables your body to regulate the glucose level in your blood. Moreover, it can release the excess fat so that you do not have much weight gain. Also, chromium is good at turning sugar into positive energy, so your cholesterol, as well as your insulin level within your body, will be kept at a safe rate. Therefore, to absorb the chromium effectively into your body, you are advised to eat more salmon, eggs, onions, turkey, broccoli, seafood, and liver.

Magnesium

Moving to the magnesium, it is crucial for your body when having diabetes. It can reduce your condition of insulin resistance where a great amount of insulin is removed by the urination process in your body.

As a result, consuming a proper amount of magnesium into your body is a great help. It can protect you from hypertension only by you eating more nuts, seeds, and vegetables, especially the green leafy types of vegetables.

Vanadium

Vanadium plays an important role in oxidating as well as transferring the glucose. Moreover, this substance can participate in helping get the glycogen into your body parts. In addition, it can prevent the glucose from being absorbed. Therefore, the metabolism process of glucose in your body will be improved.

Furthermore, you can have vanadium as a great replacement for insulin. This element can help to prevent the production of cholesterol and help you to avoid cancer. On the other hand, if you do not have enough vanadium in your body, you are more likely to have insulin resistance and diabetes.

The Powerful D

According to many types of research, most Native Americans are experiencing a deficiency of vitamin D. This condition will lead to two implications such as those in the short term and in the long term.

In terms of the short-term implications, you may have depression and the muscle pains. However, the long-term implications are more dangerous since it will lead to many serious diseases, including cancer, diabetes, and osteoporosis.

Consequently, consuming more vitamin D will help you to avoid the negative effects of type II diabetes. Thus, you can decrease the chance of insulin resistance together with endothelial dysfunction. Most of the type II diabetics are usually lacking in this vitamin, so providing more vitamin D is on the priority list when mentioning about obesity treatments.

Habitual Factors of the Vedda

There are several habitual factors that we can learn from the Vedda and directly apply to our case.

Movement
When talking about the Vedda's lifestyle, it is very proactive. More particularly, they are interested in hunting, growing crops and fishing. Therefore, they always take part in exercise instead of sitting around in one place. Therefore, one of the most effective implications is to exercise on a regular basis.

Healthy Habits
Moreover, the Vedda are very wise since they do not touch either cigarettes or other tobacco products. Furthermore, they stay away from illegal drugs as well as alcohol. Hence, to have the healthy habits like them, modern people nowadays should stay away from illegal drugs, unhealthy medication, alcohol and smoking.

Release the stress
Unlike modern busy people these days, the Vedda lives very calmly and peacefully. Therefore, they are rarely in a stressful condition. They will not have to chase after deadlines, can avoid the traffic jams and trying to pay their bills on time. As a result, you are highly recommended to put yourself in a calm and relaxing state of mind.

How to Follow these Healthy Habits to our Situation?

Exercise

To give you an overview of how to apply these principles, I am going to introduce 10 easy tips that you can remember.

1. If you want to keep yourself fit and healthy, you need to have a detailed plan on how to achieve that goal. By splitting your plan into small items and noting them down in your mind, you can always remind yourself and quickly reach that target.

2. Based on my experience, following the same schedule will make you very bored and tired. Therefore, you can change your schedule frequently by alternating the exercises every 1 week or 15 days.

4. Moreover, improving metabolism and consuming sufficient protein is a priority for diabetics. Thus, you should have a meal every 4 hours to enhance your condition. Furthermore, you should consume more carbohydrates to make yourself energetic for the whole day.

5. You need to maintain your weight effectively and have anaerobic training. By this way, your heart will be healthier.

6. Engaging in the HIIT (High-Intensity Interval Training) is considered as another amazing method to burn your excessive fat. It includes a variety of cardiovascular sessions in a continuous level. You are likely familiar with exercises such as spinning, cycling, and rowing, which fit into this category.

7. Whenever you do not want to exercise, you should not force

yourself into excessive training. Instead, you should only do a small amount of exercise such as walking on the treadmill for only 15 minutes.

Give up Smoking

You certainly know that smoking does not give you any health benefits. But you will be involved in many dangerous diseases afterward including heart attack, cancer and strokes.

In terms of diabetes, smoking will result in an unbalanced blood sugar level in your body. Moreover, it will harm your organs and the level of A1-c is going to be raised dramatically. And of course, the smokers tend to have a higher rate of this substance than the non-smokers.

Thus, I am going to show you some ultimate solutions that can help you to stop this dangerous habit.

1. Remember the good effects that giving up smoking can bring to you. Listing all the possible advantages will be the best.

2. Note down your smoking patterns every day to know the times that you are likely to smoke.

3. Firstly, choose a date when you want to eliminate smoking for an entire day and make sure to note it on the calendar.

4. Look around your house and throw all the smoking-related items away, such as the matches or the ashtrays. Moreover, you should wash your clothes carefully to get rid of the smoking smell.

5. Share your thoughts with other friends and your family member so that they can encourage your mind.

6. Make sure you exercise frequently and try to visit places that you are not allowed to smoke.

7. Drink water as much as possible to improve your hydration. Besides, don't forget to consume low-calorie foods.

Five Simple Methods to Reduce your Pressure

Exercise

You already know the stunning benefits of exercising, but we need to discuss carefully on how exercise can reduce your stress.

Based on recent studies, you can improve your focus ability and release stress related pressure by participating in a regular cardiovascular program. Also, your general wellness will be enhanced significantly. After 5 minutes of exercise, you can feel the comfort and relaxation in your body thanks to the endorphins production.

Love Yourself

Your brain is the part that controls all your internal thoughts, including the negative ideas. Consequently, you should maintain a confident mind and positive energy by always telling yourself some encouraging statements.

Go to Sleep

Sleep is regarded as one of the best options when your stress is out of your control. Everyone needs to have a proper sleep every night to be able to work properly. During your sleep, your body can repair the imbalances of chemicals and malfunctioning tissues.

However, if you cannot sleep well due to the pressure, you need to create a more comfortable environment. For example, you can lower the temperature of the air conditioner, turn off the lights and all the digital devices.

Healthy eating plan

When you are suffering from stress, you tend to eat a diversity of unhealthy foods without any notice. Hence, you should remind yourself to stay away from junk foods, as well as consume food which have more carbohydrates, fiber, and protein.

In addition, drinking coffee during your stressful condition is not a recommended solution. The reason is that the caffeine will gradually damage your nervous system.

Prepare a to-do list

Due to the modern world, you do not have much free time. Therefore, the best option is to spend about 15 minutes before your sleeping time making a plan. You should write up a detailed schedule of what you are going to do in the next few days and how to destroy your nervousness. You also need to plan your sleep accordingly to have a better sleeping quality.

Drink less alcohol

There is a large amount of ethanol contained in most of the alcoholic drinks. This substance comes from sugar and you know that a number of sweet foods can be used to make alcohol.

After drinking alcohol, your body is not able to digest it. So, most of the alcohol will be transformed into the blood vessels, as well as other body parts such as the lungs and kidneys. Then, the alcohol metabolism will begin quickly.

This process will lead to the production of toxins and tends to destroy the internal liver functions. After all, your liver will be more likely to be inflamed and contain more unhealthy fat.

Hence, you should know some effective tips for drinking less alcohol and eliminate this habit day by day:

- Throw all the alcoholic drinks inside your house away

- Choose to drink water and tea when going out with friends
- Remind yourself to drink at least 10 glasses of water daily

Body Detox

To make full use of the healthy strategies from the Vedda, you need to eliminate the toxins within your body. Thus, body detox is an incredible option for you.

Overloading of Acid

The toxins are very bad for your health and can create several unhealthy effects related to your pH levels. As you may know, if the alkaline and the acidic levels are at a proper rate inside your body, it will be the perfect situation.

Therefore, alkaline is considered as the best state for everybody. If the acid level reaches too high, you should try to remove the minerals together with the toxins from your body.

Why Should We Detox?

The reason why we should detox is to enhance our digestive system and provide more energy. Moreover, you can eliminate all the unhealthy toxins out of your body. Also, you can release the excessive fat and better your general wellness. As a result, your body will be protected from all the bad viruses and bacteria.

Detox 101

When you hear the word 'detox', it means that you are going through a process of blood cleansing. It will help to purify your liver, your skin, your lungs and your blood by getting rid of the toxins.

The Suitable Time to detox

After getting to know clearly about the benefits of detox, you should immediately plan to do it. Based on your individual needs, you need to seek out the most suitable detox schedule for yourself. For any beginners, a cleansing program in one day will be the best choice. By this way, you can reduce your stress and release the unhealthy substances out of your body.

Change your Dietary Habits

First of all, coffee and alcohol are the two things that you should keep a distance from now on. Moreover, fast foods and junk foods should be on your removal list. Furthermore, you should not consume grains, dairy foods, and meat.

Instead, you are suggested to eat foods that can cleanse your body. And my recommended list is fruits, vegetables, and seeds, along with legumes. Then, you can see my easy tips for your successful detox session below.

- Eat natural foods
- Drink a glass of hot lemon juice or eat fruits in the morning
- Consume more nuts, seeds, vegetables, fruits, and salads
- Prioritize the organic protein and Celtic salt
- Drink herbal tea
- Use coconut oil or olive oil
- Use apple vinegar to have better digestion

The 30-Day Schedule to Reduce the Sugar Level in Your Blood

Your Planned Daily Meal

According to your personal choice, you can decide what food to eat for different days. But I am going to show you a sample daily meal program for one month, so you can have a general view of what is the best to consume for yourself.

Meal	What to Eat
Breakfast	Shake, 1 egg, Salad, Vegetables
Brunch	Fruit
Lunch	Poultry, Peas, Salmon, Vegetables, Lamb
Afternoon Snack	Fruit
Dinner	Fish, Peas, Salmon, Vegetables, Poultry

Here is the detailed dietary program for a month:

Day	What to Eat	Necessary Supplements
Day 1	**One-Day Detox:** - 1 tablespoon of apple cider vinegar - 1 tablespoon of lime juice - 1 tablespoon of pure honey - 1/8 teaspoon of turmeric - 1/8 teaspoon of rosemary - 1/8 teaspoon of cayenne pepper **Fresh Fruit**	Ten 8-ounce water glasses
Day 2	- Breakfast: 2 eggs / banana / coconut milk - Lunch: Dry fruit and Mushroom - Dinner: Mushroom and Chicken Stew	• Chromium – 1000 mcg • Magnesium – 400 mg • Vitamin D – 800 IU

Day 3	- Breakfast: Mushroom Omelette - Lunch: Vegetable Soup - Dinner: Pork Stew and Apple Cider Vinegar	• Chromium – 1000 mcg • Magnesium – 400 mg • Vitamin D – 800 IU
Day 4	- Breakfast: Black Beans with Italian Sausage - Lunch: Chicken Wings with Peanut Butter - Dinner: Cranberry Meatballs	• Chromium – 1000 mcg • Magnesium – 400 mg • Vitamin D – 800 IU
Day 5	- Breakfast: Paleo Bread - Lunch: Barbeque Sausages - Dinner: Stuffed Cabbage Rolled Leaves	• Chromium – 1000 mcg • Magnesium – 400 mg • Vitamin D – 800 IU

Day 6	- Breakfast: Coconut Waffles with Almond Flour - Lunch: Honey-Rubbed Pork Wraps - Dinner: Sour and Sweet Pork	• Chromium – 1000 mcg • Magnesium – 400 mg • Vitamin D – 800 IU
Day 7	- Breakfast: Eggs Poached in Avocado - Lunch: Tuna & Salmon Muffins and Lime Sauce - Dinner: Piquant Chicken	• Chromium – 1000 mcg • Magnesium – 400 mg • Vitamin D – 800 IU
Day 8	- Breakfast: Vegetable Soup - Lunch: Barbeque Sausages - Dinner: Turkey Barbeque Wraps	• Chromium – 1000 mcg • Magnesium – 400 mg • Vitamin D – 800 IU

Day 9	- Breakfast: Almonds, Fruit and Coconut Chips - Lunch: Vegetable Soup with Beef - Dinner: Cranberry Meatballs	• Chromium – 1000 mcg • Magnesium – 400 mg • Vitamin D – 800 IU
Day 10	- Breakfast: Devilled Eggs - Lunch: Shrimp & Garlic with Coconut Milk - Dinner: Cranberry Meatballs	• Chromium – 1000 mcg • Magnesium – 400 mg • Vitamin D – 800 IU
Day 11	- Breakfast: Black Beans with Italian Sausages - Lunch: Chicken Wings with Peanut Butter - Dinner: Cranberry Meatballs	• Chromium – 1000 mcg • Magnesium – 400 mg • Vitamin D – 800 IU

Day 12	- Breakfast: Paleo Bread - Lunch: Barbeque Sausages - Dinner: Stuffed Cabbage Rolled Leaves	• Chromium – 1000 mcg • Magnesium – 400 mg • Vitamin D – 800 IU
Day 13	- Breakfast: Coconut Waffles with Almond Flour - Lunch: Honey-Rubbed Pork Wraps - Dinner: Sour and Sweet Pork	• Chromium – 1000 mcg • Magnesium – 400 mg • Vitamin D – 800 IU
Day 14	- Breakfast: Poached Eggs with Avocado - Lunch: Tuna & Salmon Muffins and Lime Sauce - Dinner: Piquant Chicken	• Chromium – 1000 mcg • Magnesium – 400 mg • Vitamin D – 800 IU

Day 15	- Breakfast: Vegetable Soup - Lunch: Barbeque Sausages - Dinner: Turkey Barbeque Wraps	• Chromium – 1000 mcg • Magnesium – 400 mg • Vitamin D – 800 IU
Day 16	- Breakfast: Devilled Eggs - Lunch: Shrimp & Garlic with Coconut Milk - Dinner: Cranberry Meatballs	• Chromium – 1000 mcg • Magnesium – 400 mg • Vitamin D – 800 IU
Day 17	- Breakfast: Mushroom Omelette - Lunch: Vegetable Soup - Dinner: Pork Stew and Apple Cider Vinegar	• Chromium – 1000 mcg • Magnesium – 400 mg • Vitamin D – 800 IU

Day 18	- Breakfast: Black Beans with Italian Sausages - Lunch: Chicken Wings with Peanut Butter - Dinner: Cranberry Meatballs	• Chromium – 1000 mcg • Magnesium – 400 mg • Vitamin D – 800 IU
Day 19	- Breakfast: Coconut Flakes, Raisins and Walnuts - Lunch: Barbeque Sausages - Dinner: Stuffed Cabbage Rolled Leaves	• Chromium – 1000 mcg • Magnesium – 400 mg • Vitamin D – 800 IU
Day 20	- Breakfast: Coconut Waffles with Almond Flour - Lunch: Honey-Rubbed Pork Wraps - Dinner: Sour and Sweet Pork	• Chromium – 1000 mcg • Magnesium – 400 mg • Vitamin D – 800 IU

Day 21	- Breakfast: Poached Eggs with Avocado - Lunch: Tuna & Salmon Muffins and Lime Sauce - Dinner: Piquant Chicken	• Chromium – 1000 mcg • Magnesium – 400 mg • Vitamin D – 800 IU
Day 22	- Breakfast: Vegetable Soup - Lunch: Barbeque Sausages - Dinner: Turkey Barbeque Wraps	• Chromium – 1000 mcg • Magnesium – 400 mg • Vitamin D – 800 IU
Day 23	- Breakfast: Devilled Eggs - Lunch: Shrimp & Garlic with Coconut Milk - Dinner: Cranberry Meatballs	• Chromium – 1000 mcg • Magnesium – 400 mg • Vitamin D – 800 IU

Day 24	- Breakfast: Mushroom Omelette - Lunch: Vegetable Soup - Dinner: Pork Stew and Apple Cider Vinegar	• Chromium – 1000 mcg • Magnesium – 400 mg • Vitamin D – 800 IU
Day 25	- Breakfast: Black Beans with Italian Sausages - Lunch: Chicken Wings with Peanut Butter - Dinner: Cranberry Meatballs	• Chromium – 1000 mcg • Magnesium – 400 mg • Vitamin D – 800 IU
Day 26	- Breakfast: Coconut Flakes, Raisins and Walnuts - Lunch: Barbeque Sausages - Dinner: Stuffed Cabbage Rolled Leaves	• Chromium – 1000 mcg • Magnesium – 400 mg • Vitamin D – 800 IU

Day 27	- Breakfast: Coconut Waffles and Almond Flour - Lunch: Honey-Rubbed Pork Wraps - Dinner: Sour and Sweet Pork	• Chromium – 1000 mcg • Magnesium – 400 mg • Vitamin D – 800 IU
Day 28	- Breakfast: Poached Eggs with Avocado - Lunch: Tuna & Salmon Muffins and Lime Sauce - Dinner: Piquant Chicken	• Chromium – 1000 mcg • Magnesium – 400 mg • Vitamin D – 800 IU
Day 29	- Breakfast: Vegetable Soup - Lunch: Barbeque Sausages - Dinner: Turkey Barbeque Wraps	• Chromium – 1000 mcg • Magnesium – 400 mg • Vitamin D – 800 IU
Day 30	- Breakfast: Devilled Eggs - Lunch: Shrimp & Garlic with Coconut Milk - Dinner: Cranberry Meatballs	• Chromium – 1000 mcg • Magnesium – 400 mg • Vitamin D – 800 IU

Detailed recipes and instruction for the above program

Mushroom Omelet

Ingredients:

- 1 cup of chopped mushrooms
- 2 teaspoons of nondairy milk
- ½ cup of egg beaters
- 1 teaspoon of olive oil
- 1 dash of pepper
- 1 dash of salt

Instructions

You can use the olive oil to stir-fry the mushrooms until they become softer. It is estimated to take at least 5 minutes. Then, you can create a mixture of pepper, olive oil, salt, milk and some eggs. Make sure to combine this mixture by using the heated skillet. When everything is set after cooking for 4 minutes, you can put the mushrooms into this mixture and continue to stir-fry for 3 minutes.

You can turn the opposite side of the omelet only by using the spatula. Finally, you can eat this dish with the vegetables.

Black Beans with Italian Sausages

Ingredients

- 12 oz, of chopped Italian sausage
- ½ chopped onion
- ½ cup of black beans
- ½ cup of tomato puree
- 1½ cup of minced green chilies
- 2 basil leaves
- 1 teaspoon of pepper

- ¾ tablespoon of salt
- 1 teaspoon of vegetable oil

Instructions

First, you need to combine the chilies and onions together. After that, don't forget to sauté them with the olive oil in 4 minutes. Then, you can pour the remaining ingredients into the pot and leave them to cook for 3 hours.

Devilled Eggs

Ingredients

- 6 hard-boiled eggs
- ¼ cup of pureed avocado
- 1 dash of black pepper
- 2 teaspoons of vinegar
- 1 dash of salt

Instructions

You need to cut all 6 eggs into halves and remember to put the yolks aside. Then, you can combine the yolks with the other items and mix them together. After the mixture is quite smooth, you can divide it into equal portions, put it back inside the eggs and have your meal.

Coconut Flakes with Walnut Raisins

Ingredients

- ¼ cup of walnuts
- ¼ cups of raisins
- ½ cup of sugar-free coconut chips or flakes

Instructions

Use the bowl to store all the ingredients and then pour the nondairy milk into this bowl.

Poached Eggs with Avocado

Ingredients

- 3 avocados
- 3 eggs

Instructions

You are advised to poach these 3 eggs based on your personal preference. After that, you can put them into the avocados and serve yourself.

Vegetable Soup

Ingredients

- Celery
- Yellow squash
- Leeks
- Garlic
- Vegetable broth
- Oregano
- Salt
- Green beans
- Zucchini
- Red peppers
- Onions
- Shredded cabbage
- Basil

Instructions

After buying all the vegetables above, you need to cut and mix them together in a pot except for the vegetable broth. The reason is that you need to heat the vegetable broth before putting them into this mixture. Then, you can cook all of them in a total of 15 minutes. Lastly, you can put the oregano, the salt, as well as the basil for a better taste.

Chicken Wings with Peanut Butter

Ingredients

- 5 chicken wings
- 1 teaspoon of salt
- 1 cup of water
- 3 tablespoons of peanut butter
- 1 tablespoon of ground ginger

Instructions

This recipe is very simple since you only need to put everything together into the cooker. Then, you can leave them on the stove for about 5 hours until you see that they are soft enough.

Dry Fruit and Mushroom

Ingredients

- ½ cup of button mushrooms
- 2 cups of chopped almonds
- 1 cup of chopped cashews
- 2 cardamom cloves
- 1 chopped onion
- 2 garlic cloves
- 1 teaspoon of salt
- 1 teaspoon of olive oil
- 1 cup of water

Instructions

With this recipe, you need to use the cooker again. Make sure to sauté the onions and the garlic cloves until you see a brown color. At this stage, you can add all the rest to the cooker and wait for an additional 7 hours to serve yourself.

Barbeque Sausages

Ingredients

- 1 chopped onion
- 12 oz. of smoked sausages
- 2 tablespoons of apple cider vinegar
- ½ teaspoon of paprika powder
- 1 teaspoon of salt
- 1 teaspoon of cayenne pepper
- ½ cup of water
- 1 teaspoon of olive oil

Instructions

With this food, you can make use of the slow cooker. You should sauté the onions first. Then, you can cook it with the rest for 5 hours.

Honey-Rubbed Pork Wraps

Ingredients

- 12 oz. of boneless pork
- 1 chopped onion
- ½ cup of water
- 2 tablespoons of Worcestershire sauce
- ¼ cup of tomato puree
- 1 teaspoon of garlic ginger paste
- 2 tablespoons of honey
- 1 teaspoon of salt
- Lettuce leaves

Instructions

All the ingredients above except the lettuce should be mixed together in the slow cooker for about 12 hours.

Shrimp & Garlic with Coconut Milk

Ingredients

- 12 oz. of peeled shrimp
- 1 tablespoon of olive oil
- 4 garlic cloves
- ¾ cup of coconut milk
- 1 teaspoon of lemon juice
- Coriander leaves
- 1 teaspoon of salt

Instructions

Again, with the slow cooker, you can sauté the garlic in the olive oil. After that, you can cook the rest with this mixture for 5 hours.

Mushroom and Chicken Stew

Ingredients

- 1 lb. of chicken breasts
- ½ cup of button mushrooms
- 2 sliced celery stalks
- 1 teaspoon of salt
- ¼ cup of red wine
- 2 garlic cloves
- ½ cup of tomato puree

Instructions

Make sure to combine these ingredients and cook them in the slow cooker for at least 6 hours.

Pork Stew and Apple Cider Vinegar

Ingredients

- 1 lb. of pork roast

- 2 tablespoons of apple cider vinegar
- ½ cup of sweet potato
- 1 teaspoon of thyme
- 1 teaspoon of parsley
- 1 teaspoon of salt
- 1 cup of water

Instructions

This food is prepared by combining all the ingredients together. And then, you can put all of them into the slow cooker and cook for 7 hours.

Sour and Sweet Pork

Ingredients

- 4 pork chops
- 1½ cups of diced carrots
- 1½ cups of broccoli florets
- 10 oz. of chopped pineapple
- 1 bell pepper
- 2½ tablespoons of Worcestershire sauce
- 2 tablespoons of vinegar
- ½ teaspoon of salt

Instructions

For this food, you need to keep the pineapple aside and put all the other ingredients into a large pot. Then, you can leave them on the stove for 7 hours before adding the pineapples.

Piquant Chicken

Ingredients

- 1 lb. of chopped chicken
- 1 chopped onion
- 2 garlic cloves
- 1½ tablespoons of curry powder

- 1 teaspoon of apple cider vinegar
- 6 raisins
- 5 almonds
- ½ cup of tomato puree

Instructions

You can serve this wonderful dish by sautéing the onions and the bell peppers first. Then, put all the remaining items together and cook for 7 hours.

I. CHAPTER III. HIIT – THE WEAPON TO FIGHT DIABETES

What is HIIT?

Talking about the HIIT, it stands for the High-Intensity Interval Training, which is an improved program with many short-time sessions of anaerobic exercise. Moreover, you can think about it as a cardiovascular workout program. Apart from HIIT, there are two other names for this program, including the Sprint Interval Training (SIT) or High-Intensity Intermittent Exercise (HIIE).

A normal HIIT session is between 5 to 30 minutes depending on your ability. These sessions will support your athletic capacity, as well as improve your health condition.

How HIIT Works

In general, HIIT sessions will force your muscles to have more active movement than the other types of programs. Therefore, your body can enhance the response of insulin, as well as decrease the glycogen level of the muscles. In the end, you can achieve the goal of triggering insulin production better.

If you used to participating in the HIIT sessions, you will know that they include diverse intense physical activities. You can start with warm-up exercises and then do the intense programs on a repeated basis.

Furthermore, you can have the medium intense exercises to suit your condition. These exercises aim to help you recover from the extremely intense exercises.

Not all the exercises included in HIIT are the same. They are different in length and frequency, but you are highly recommended to do the highly intense exercises at least 20 seconds and repeat it three consecutive times. For the best result, you should have a personal trainer consulting the suitable level of exercise intensity to you. By doing this, you can have the most proper exercises which are suitable for your age, your medical condition, along with your gender.

Types of HIIT Regimens

These days, HIIT is created with many different versions, but Peter Coe was the first one to develop this incredible program in the world. Hence, to reduce your confusion, I am going to show you the most common programs of HIIT.

The Peter Coe Protocol

As I mentioned above, Peter Coe was the first one to develop HIIT, so he was very well-known in the 1970s. He created a specific training with high impact and many recovery intervals. The particular exercise that he used to have was repetitions of 200-meter races. Between the races, there will be some recovery periods of 30 seconds in total.

The Tabata Regimen

Going to the next one, the Tabata Regimen has earned the popularity of being the next effective HIIT version. This program was designed by Izuma Tabata, who used to be an Olympic speed skater as well as a professor. His training consists of a set of intense exercises in 20 seconds and many intervals in 10 seconds. You need to do this exercise repeatedly in 4 minutes.

This set of intense programs is called as IE1 Protocol. Many athletes follow this exercise about 4 times a week and they can achieve the same results as those who apply it 5 times. As a result, more and more people are keen on this intense protocol since they desire to burn more fat as well as lower the risks of having diabetes.

The Gibala Regimen

This protocol will remind you about Martin Gibala who is a professor at a university. He and his colleagues used to spend much time researching the HIIT exercises. Therefore, he started creating a new version which is a combination of warm-up sessions and intense exercise. You need to get started in 3 minutes, and then take part in the intense training in an hour with some 75-second resting parts. Also, it is important to repeat this process at least 12 times.

I have to say that Gibala Protocol is quite challenging, but it is very effective for your overall wellness. However, if your physical condition is not suitable for this extremely intense program, you can choose the less intense one. This is considered as the lighter option for anyone who always stays at one place without exercising in a long time.

Especially, this training program includes the warm-up session, the repetition of exercises and the recovery periods. You can have 3 minutes to get heated, 1 minutes to exercise and 1 minute to relax in the middle. At last, the protocol completes with the cooling-down intervals, which will take you 5 minutes.

The Timmons Protocol

Next, I am going to introduce the final HIIT version that will capture your attention. Designed by Jamie Timmons, the Timmons protocol is the combination of three sets of biking and one set of cycling. In particular, you can ride the bike for 2 minutes and finish with 20 seconds of cycling.

However, you should keep in mind that regularly exercising will help you a lot. Keep practicing at least 3 times a week and maintain 20 minutes for each session. If you keep this habit, your body sensitivity to insulin will be much improved and will burn the extra fat in your body faster.

The Reasons Why People Follow HIIT

An increased number of obese people are interested in following HIIT. Do you know the reasons?

First of all, this training program is divided into many different versions all over the world. As a result, it is ideal and easy to follow regardless of your age, your physical condition or your fitness level. Furthermore, you cannot deny its benefits of burning fat quickly and helping to prevent the development of diabetes.

Besides, HIIT protocols are very diverse for people of all ages and all skills. According to your personal interest, you can take part in the suitable programs such as swimming, walking, cycling, as well as aqua training. So, this workout is very flexible.

Also, you can be trained regularly and extremely to have a good health. After all, you can increase your endurance in a short time. Instead of the normal way of exercising, applying HIIT exercises will help you burn more fat and calories.

The Relationship between HIIT and Diabetes

Nowadays, more people are involved with diabetes and obesity. We do not know why this disease has appeared more in the world and caused a number of deaths.

As a consequence, we need to stop this negative condition by following the right and proper methods. And with no doubt, HIIT is famous for being one of the most reliable and effective protocols to cure type II diabetes in the world. Next, we are going to focus on how HIIT works to prevent the development of diabetes for people.

How Can HIIT Cure Type II Diabetes?

Based on many researchers, HIIT exercises are reported to be able to reduce the glucose level efficiently. In addition, it is very effective for giving you some quick improvements for anyone enduring cardiovascular diseases, as well as the type II diabetes. In particular, your heartbeat rate tends to rise a lot when you conduct this intense training.

During this period, more blood will be pumped into the necessary internal organs, which provides them with more oxygen. Thanks to this procedure, the metabolism process will be enhanced greatly, and you can control your blood sugar better. Furthermore, the intense workouts are very excellent at protecting you from getting the cardiovascular diseases and diabetes as well.

Useful Tips to Have an Effective HIIT Training Exercises

Many people find HIIT training program extremely challenging and daunting, so they tend to lose the energy, the motivation and the interest in participating in this program for a long time.

As a consequence, I am willing to share some of my useful tips that can bring back your motivation and keep you from giving up this healthy habit.

1. **Do not hurry to start.** You need to take some time to get used to this challenging training program because your physical condition cannot endure the extremely intense exercise from the beginning. Therefore, you can start off slowly and then increase

the intensity level gradually when you feel that your body can totally get familiar with these workouts.

For instance, you can get started with the light cardio exercises, cycling or running in 15 minutes. As time passes, you can increase the duration of this exercise according to your physical ability.

2. **Choose your favorite workouts first.** For the beginners, I highly advise that you should choose the exercises that you have the most interest in. Although it is going to burn fewer calories than the other workouts, it is a wise choice to maintain your routines for a longer time.

You should never choose the ones that you hate since you will gradually lose your motivation during the intervals. And of course, it is not the way you are going to do it, so it is important to choose your favorites.

3. **Add sufficient energy to your body.** When you conduct the intense program for a while, you are able to burn more calories since the intensity level will be increased a lot. But many people are trying to eat less and less to keep their weight reduced. And this is not a smart thing to do.

Skipping meals and letting yourself feel hungry will make your body weaker and more tired. Therefore, your body cannot do the intense programs to stimulate the metabolism system and then eliminate the excessive fat. As a result, keeping a proper dietary plan with sufficient protein and carbohydrates will be needed to give your body adequate energy.

4. **Have a timer.** Make sure that you care about the time whenever you do the intervals during your training. It is very important since you can keep track of when to start the exercise, when to stop and when to change the exercises. Moreover, you can control the movement of your performance and give yourself an overview of the time required for each exercise.

Based on my real-life experience, you cannot focus on the time unless you have the timer. Thus, you tend to either relax more or exercise more than you should. A number of people have this problem and it will greatly destroy their training program.

Hence, keep in mind that you should always bring along a timer to reach the best results after each training session.

5. **Focus on your physical condition.** Many people make a mistake when they always force themselves to do the difficult exercises to burn as much fat as possible from the start. However, you should listen to your body. If you go beyond your body limit, you may make your body injured and hurt without any notice. As a consequence, you are recommended to select the suitable workouts for your body. By doing this, you can have a happy and encouraging training time.

6. **Get familiar with various exercises.** If you have a personal trainer, he will tell you to follow a certain set of exercises which are the most suitable to your state. But you should sometimes change to the other workouts since it will be more interesting. Following the same exercises for a long time will make you bored and tired, leading to a decrease in the motivation. So, do not hesitate to replace some of your exercises with swimming, running or cycling.

7. **Do not extend your session more than 1 minute.** You may think that you can endure the intense session for more than 60 seconds. It is true, but it means that you are not putting all of your efforts into the exercises. You have to become totally exhausted after any sessions since it means that all of the necessary parts of your body are truly working.

8. **Do not go less than 10 seconds for tough exercise.** As I mentioned before, you should not go over 60 seconds and this time, you should endure at least 10 seconds even for the tough exercises. If you cannot achieve this requirement, you have to do more cycle to have the best results.

9. **Have a good recovery process.** Recovery is always a good step when your muscles are totally exhausted after hard training.

Therefore, you need to give yourself enough time to recover and have energy again. Your muscles will need to rest and relax for the next training.

10. **Focus on timing yourself.** Do not neglect this crucial step. You can get incredible benefits from timing yourself. You can have yourself obey the duration when focusing on the time every session and interval.

11. **Remember to have proper intervals even for the lowly intense session.** Many people are wrong when thinking they can ignore the intervals when they can endure the sessions. Regardless of the low or high intensity, you have to proceed with the planned intervals to have the best resting periods. These intervals are designed to help you refill your stamina, lower the blood sugar and burn the excessive calories.

12. **Seek professional advice from the doctors.** After deciding to go for any training protocol, you should meet your doctor at first. These programs are designed for anyone in general, but it is a wise decision to ask for a professional opinion before really getting started. You will not lose anything but will have more courage to start your chosen program for a long time.

13. **Record your heart rate, your glucose level, and your blood pressure.** Before you start this long-time program, you should keep a record of your body. Moreover, you should repeat this step during and after your exercises. By updating these figures regularly, you can know the improvements in your condition. Otherwise, you can know how to reverse your problems better.

14. **Get your necessary medication**. After meeting your doctor, you may be required to take some drugs for diabetes. You need to follow the instructions of your doctor and do not stop them unless your doctor advises. If your doctor really permits you, you can stop taking the medication during your HIIT training.

Blood Sugar Lowering Smoothies

I know what you're thinking: the Vedda people of Sri Lanka don't actually drink smoothies!

You're right, but smoothies happen to be a delicious, convenient way to include special ingredients from the Vedda diet into your daily routine and give your body a power-packed energy boost. Better still, each mouthful will be helping you to a diabetes-free future.

Our smoothies will give you all of the nutrients you need in one easy-to-consume meal.

In addition to the specific nutrients that we've identified as being beneficial for your diabetes, improving intake of green vegetables in general is a great way to improve your overall health. This goes counter to what we see in society at large.

1. Coconut Berry Whip

Ingredients:

- ¾ cup So Delicious strawberry cultured coconut milk

- ½ cup light coconut milk

- ½ cup fresh raspberries

Procedures:

Combine all of the ingredients in a blender and blend until smooth. Divide between two glasses and serve, or store in the refrigerator for three to four days.

2. Avocado Coconut Squeeze

Ingredients:

- 1 frozen banana

- 1 avocado, pitted and peeled

- 1 ½ cups coconut milk

- 1 teaspoon honey

- 1-ounce dark chocolate, shaved

Procedures:

Combine all of the ingredients in a blender and blend until smooth.

Divide between two glasses and serve immediately.

3. Super Berry Smoothie

Ingredients:

- ½ cup frozen raspberries
- ½ cup frozen blueberries
- ½ cup 100 percent tart cherry juice
- ¼ cup water
- ¼ cup nondairy yogurt
- ½ cup coconut milk
- 1 teaspoon honey (optional)

Procedures:

Combine the coconut milk, berries, cherry juice, and water in a blender and blend until icy and smooth. Add the yogurt and blend. If desired, sweeten with honey. Divide between two glasses and serve, or store in the refrigerator for three to four days.

4. Hemp Shake

Ingredients:

¾ cup nondairy yogurt

1 banana

½ cup almond milk

1 tablespoon hemp powder 4 or

5 ice cubes

1 teaspoons honey (optional)

Procedures:

Combine the yogurt, banana, almond milk, and hemp powder in a blender and blend until smooth. Add the ice cubes and honey (if desired) and blend until frothy. Divide between two glasses and serve, or store in the refrigerator for three to four days.

5. Cinnamon Swirl

Ingredients:

- 1 cup nondairy yogurt
- ½ cup coconut milk
- ½ cup raisins
- 1 teaspoon ground cinnamon

4 or 5 ice cubes

Procedures:

Combine the yogurt, milk, and raisins in a blender and blend until smooth. Add the cinnamon and ice and blend again until smooth. Divide between two glasses and serve, or store in the refrigerator for three to four days.

6. Strawberry Spinach Power

Ingredients:

- 1½ cups nondairy yogurt
- 5 strawberries
- ½ cup packed baby spinach
- 4 or 5 ice cubes

Procedures:

Combine all of the ingredients in a blender and blend until smooth.

Divide between two glasses and serve, or store in the refrigerator for three to four days.

7. Raspberry Ginger Slush

Ingredients:

- 1 cup frozen raspberries
- 1 cup ginger beer
- ½ cup water

Procedures:

Combine the raspberries, ginger beer, and water in a blender and blend until icy and smooth. Divide between two glasses and serve.

8. *Orange Banana Smoothie*

Ingredients:

- 1 banana

- 2 tablespoons water

- 1 cup 100 percent orange juice

Procedures:

Combine the banana and water in a blender and blend until smooth. Add the orange juice and blend until combined. Divide between two glasses and serve, or store in the refrigerator for three to four days.

9. Fruit Punch Smoothie

Ingredients:

- ¾ cup So Delicious strawberry cultured coconut milk
- 2 kiwis, peeled
- 1 banana
- 1 cup frozen sweet dark cherries
- ½ cup nondairy milk
- ¼ cup 100 percent white grape juice

Procedures:

Combine all of the ingredients in a blender and blend until icy and smooth. Divide between two glasses and serve, or store in the refrigerator for three to four days.

10. Silky Coco Smoothie

Ingredients:

- 1½ cups unsweetened coconut milk beverage (such as from So Delicious)
- 1 avocado, pitted and peeled
- 1 tablespoon unsweetened cocoa powder
- 1 tablespoon agave nectar

Procedures:

Combine ½ cup of the coconut milk with the avocado in a blender and blend until smooth.

Add the remaining 1 cup coconut milk, cocoa powder, and agave nectar and blend again, until smooth.

Divide between two glasses and serve.

11. *Butternut Squash Smoothie*

Ingredients:

- ½ cup sliced leeks
- 1 cup chilled roasted butternut squash
- 1 cup vegetable broth
- ¼ teaspoon garlic powder
- 1/8 teaspoon sea salt

Procedures:

Heat a small skillet over medium heat. Add the sliced leeks to the dry pan and cook, stirring, until tender, about five to seven minutes.

Combine the sautéed leeks, squash, broth, and garlic powder in a blender and blend until smooth. If the mixture is too thick, add water to thin it to the desired consistency. Finish with the sea salt. Serve, or store in the refrigerator for three to four days.

12. Banana Berry Smoothie

Ingredients:

- ½ banana

- 4 to 5 strawberries, hulled

- ½ cup almond milk

- ¼ cup 100 percent orange juice

- 1 teaspoon agave nectar

Procedures:

Combine the banana, strawberries, almond milk, orange juice, and agave nectar in a blender. Add the ice cubes and blend to combine. Serve, or store in the refrigerator for three to four days.

13. Berry Beet Smoothie

Ingredients:

- 1 cup nondairy milk

- 1 cup sliced strawberries

- 1 small beet, peeled

- 1 to 2 teaspoons agave nectar (optional)

Procedures:

Combine the milk, strawberries, and beet in a blender and blend until smooth.

Taste, and add agave nectar if desired.

Serve, or store in the refrigerator for three to four days.

14. Clean Breeze Smoothie

Ingredients:

2 ripe and peeled kiwis

½ cup nondairy yogurt

6 ice cubes

1 small cucumber, chopped

1 cup kombucha, ginger-flavored

2 tablespoons fresh cilantro leaves

Procedures:

Blend cucumber, kiwi, and kombucha. Then add the yogurt and the cilantro. Finally, blend in the 6 ice cubes until the smoothie becomes frothy and smooth.

Serve.

15. Antioxidant Smoothie

Ingredients:

- 1 cup pomegranate juice, fresh and unsweetened
- 2 cups frozen mixed berries
- 1 cup water

Procedures:

Blend all ingredients until frothy and smooth. Serve.

16. Mango Coconut Smoothie

Ingredients:

- ¾ cup mango, frozen

- ½ cup coconut milk

- 1 tablespoon chia seeds

- 1 teaspoon nutmeg, ground

- 2 tablespoons coconut, shredded and unsweetened

Procedures:

Blend frozen mango with coconut milk until smooth. While blending, add in chia seeds, shredded coconut, and nutmeg. Pour in a glass and serve.

17. Soothing Smoothie

Ingredients:

- 1 ripe banana
- 2 tablespoons maple syrup
- 1 cup strong chamomile tea
- 1 cup nondairy yogurt

Procedures:

Pour the chamomile tea into an ice cube tray and place the tray in the freezer to freeze. Blend ripe banana, maple syrup and yogurt. When chamomile tea is frozen, add the cubes into the blender and blend until smooth.

18. Channel Orange Smoothie

Ingredients:

- 1 red bell pepper, quartered

- 1 navel orange, peeled

- 1 tablespoon coconut oil

- 1 teaspoon cayenne pepper or cinnamon, ground

Procedures:

Blend red bell pepper, orange, and coconut oil. While blending, add cayenne pepper or cinnamon.

Continue bending until smooth and then serve immediately afterwards.

19. Coconut Boost Smoothie

Ingredients:

- 1 cup nondairy yogurt
- 3 tablespoons orange juice, fresh
- 1 cup pure coconut water, chilled
- 1 cup mango chunks, fresh and frozen
- 2 cubes ice

Procedures:

Blend all ingredients until smooth. Serve.

20. Yogurt Mint Smoothie

Ingredients:

- 1 cup nondairy yogurt
- 1 cup cubed cucumber
- 2 tablespoons fresh mint
- 1 tablespoon fresh lemon juice
- 1 teaspoon garlic powder

Procedures:

Combine all the ingredients in a blender and blend until smooth. Divide between two glasses and serve, or store in the refrigerator for three to four days.

V. CONCLUSION

Any diabetics will have a hope to get rid of diabetes as soon as possible. You are considered as a patient for a long time and it is time for you to get up.

My sharing in terms of the healthy habit and lifestyle of the Vedda, it will help you to quickly get out of this terrible condition. By following the dietary plan as well as the HIIT training, you can remove the diabetes effects from your life permanently.

If your dream comes true, you will never have to meet the doctors for advice, have the injections, avoid your favorite foods and always feel worried about your health condition. Going through this book will raise your hope and provide you the motivation to live a healthy life. Thanks for reading until the end and I wish all the best for you!

Thank you again!

I really wish that you can enjoy my sharing and knowledge!

Lastly, please do not hesitate to write me your thoughts about my book since I really appreciate your idea. However, in case you have any confusion and queries, please feel free to keep in touch with me anytime.